HOMEMADE HAND SANITIZER

A Best and Simple Step-By-Step Guide on How to Make Your Anti-Bacterial Hand Sanitizer to Protect from Infections caused by Viruses and Germs.

(Best Author of "HOMEMADE FACE MASK")

STEVEN GRAY

Table of Contents

INTRODUCTION

Hand sanitizer is a fluid, spray, or gel widely used on hands to decrease viruses and bacteria. Handwashing with soap and water is usually preferred in most environments and it cannot extract harmful chemicals unlike soap and water. People can wipe away the hand sanitizer incorrectly before it has been dried, and some are quite useful because the concentrations of alcohol are too low.

Hand sanitizers based on alcohol are superior in most health-care environments to hand washing with soap and water. Reasons include being treated better and being more effective. Hand washing with soap and water only can be done if contamination can be observed, or after use of the toilet, it should be done.

Usually, alcohol-based versions contain a mixture of isopropyl alcohol, ethanol (ethyl alcohol), or n-propanol, with the most effective versions containing 60 to 95 per cent alcohol. Care should be taken because it is flame-retardant. Hand sanitizer based with alcohol protects against a large variety of microorganisms but not spores. Compounds like glycerol can be added to avoid skin drying. Many variants contain fragrances; however, due to the possibility of allergic reactions these are discouraged. Non-alcoholic versions typically contain benzalkonium chloride or triclosan; however, they are less effective than alcoholic versions.

ABOUT THIS GUIDE

This guide is all about the Homemade Hand Sanitizer and it is unique from all of the others. The way the guideline is designed makes it easier to find the solution you are looking for. Go ahead and click the Guide to see for yourself. Nice bold headings direct your eyes to only the section you like, and you do not have to read the whole text for a quick response. This guide offers an exhaustive description of all facets of DIY your Hand Sanitizer at home. Need details about how to get started? Here is the description too. So, place this tutorial up on your bookcase in a prominent spot. We are confident you will go back to that again and again.

DIY HOMEMADE HAND
SANITIZER ALCOHOL FREE

This Homemade Hand Sanitizer is incredibly cheap and easy to make and also non-toxic!

Important Note: Prior using a home remedy, every time supervision of a health care provider is necessary, as this has never been checked in a laboratory. Also, this hand sanitizer formulation does not have the sixty percent + alcohol level required by the CDC and other medical associations for hand sanitizer to combat against virus effectively.

Everybody has never been a hand sanitizer fan; you know the common kind all around dispensers! someone has had delicate skin and they just don't comply with them. In reality, whenever someone has had to use these, their skin fissures, and bleeds everywhere within hours. And when they took a course on food standards, they told us that proper usage and methods of hand washing are much more productive.

How to make hand sanitizer without alcohol?

You should use Witch Hazel instead of alcohol as the basis and is better for fighting off germs. It might not be as strong as Vodka claims, but it does some good! Moreover, many individuals who choose to use a handmade hand sanitizer for kids tend to use Witch Hazel as a basis instead of alcohol. You might also want to check out the plant therapy blend of Germ Buster

Essential Oils which is designed for babies. Not all the essential oils are mostly safe for kids, so it's nice to have a mixture made up already.

Why use alcohol as a base rather than Witch Hazel?

In destroying most germs, alcohol such as isopropyl (rubbing alcohol) is very efficient. Witch hazel is productive but not so much. Research says that 60-90% of alcohol is safer, which seems fairly decent. Particularly when you're talking about moving from the plane to the rental cars.

Why to make your own hand sanitizer?

It's non-toxic There are some strong brands to be purchased in quality food shops on the market. But the regular grocery store products are replete with harmful chemicals.

Cost – Making your own hand sanitizer is very economically viable, and also super easy. We can produce a batch in just a few minutes lasting for months.

Sensitive skin – Those who have very sensitive skin, so the sanitizer must be made by considering the sensitivity of the skin.

Traveling – That kind of never even needs a description! It's super convenient and have something to destroy off germs even when you are travelling.

Cold and flu season – Although alcohol is not 100

percent efficient for all pathogens, isopropyl alcohol is 99.9% successful for non-spore - forming bacteria and combats several other viruses and seasonal flu.

What to store your hand sanitizer in?

Any squeeze or little bottle of spray that you have. The 2 you see pictured here used to be store hand sanitizer bottles. In shops you can also verify the trip bottle category, while these types of bottles are not as excellent quality and will be leaked over time. REI also has a great selection of small containers that are useful for homemade bath & body brands to start taking backpacking.

Try using an opaque dark colored bottle to protect essential oils, if you can spot one, (they are prone to light). Obviously, you have not to be concerned a lot about this, because these hand sanitizer bottles can remain in a dark for long.

What essential oils are best for homemade hand sanitizer?

Lemon essential oil – Antiseptic properties, disinfectants, and antifungals.

Lavender essential oil – Anti-bacterial, antiviral, and I also love that smell!

Tea Tree essential oil – Anti-fungal, antimicrobial, antiseptic, antiviral, and antibacterial – whew... that's a lot!

Others to consider – There are also antibacterial effects of eucalyptus, clove, cinnamon, lime, peppermint, rosemary, herb, and garlic.

Steps

An easy way to use non-toxic hand sanitizer suitable for both traveling and running errands!

INGREDIENTS

For a spray bottle:

- 3 Tablespoons Aloe Vera gel

- 3 Tablespoons witch hazel, isopropyl alcohol, ethanol, or vodka

- 15 drops lemon essential oil

- 15 drops lavender essential oil

- 15–30 drops of tea tree essential oil, see notes

For a squeeze bottle:

- 1/4 cup Aloe Vera gel

- 2 Tablespoons witch hazel, isopropyl alcohol, ethanol, or vodka

- 15 drops lemon essential oil

- 15 drops lavender essential oil

- 15–30 drops of tea tree essential oil, see notes

INSTRUCTIONS

Mix all the ingredients together either for the recycle spray or squeeze bottle. You can do this by bringing them specifically into your tank through a funnel. Or you can blend them together in a small pot, then drain them into your selected jar (or very cautiously).

If you are using a glass bottle, make sure to keep it in a dark position to better protect the essential oils' qualities. Essential oils can segregate over time, and before every use, you must shake up your hand sanitizer.

NOTES

The more oil you use for tea tree, the more efficient it is

in preventing infections. Honestly, however, someone have some intolerances to this specific oil, so use the minimal quantity that appears to work great for skin. These are often commonly considered to be healthy oils for most users, as an essential oil safeguard. However, bear in mind that they do not work for you and if you have any effects at all, you can still receive advice from a health practitioner / abandon using them! In certain cases, any of these oils can also have a photosensitivity where you will get a discomfort when the skin is exposed to the light.

DIY Hand Sanitizer Spray (Alcohol-free and Kid-Safe)

Everyone must start making their own DIY items because we are all worried about common toxics. Since these collect in our bodies, everybody's chief concern is toxic chemicals and endocrine disruptors, and they have been associated with all kinds of ailments alongside cancer. It makes you question if all of the cancer that surrounds us is relevant to everything, we 're prone to.

We have to make it a mission to reduce our children's exposure to toxic chemicals, and one of the best ways to do so when you make your own DIY products.
That way, you know exactly what's in everything. For this we have to   know that the ingredients are clean, and we don't have to use preservatives because we have to make them in small quantities.

Hand sanitizer is one of the items we have to keep in our diaper bag.   Ideally, we 'd always clean our hands with proper soap and water but that isn't always possible, and this is where hand sanitizer fits in.

What's wrong with hand sanitizers?
Some sanitizers have additives which we have to avoid within our family. Here are the major concerns:

Triclosan: Is used in cosmetic products as bactericide. The concern with this is it helps to create antibiotic resistant bacteria and has been related to degradation of hormone activity.

Fragrances: The issue with this is that corporations are not forced to reveal what is in their scents and much of the time the chemicals used to make them include phthalates and parabens-both endocrine disruptors.

Alcohol: This is one of the most essential components in hand sanitizer and the logic they smell the way they do. The trouble with that is that it might be dangerous for them if your child were to consume it – and things like that happened. As for other kinds of alcohols being used hand sanitizers, there are several other questions too.

Hand sanitizer should NOT replace hand washing

This may sound like rational thinking, but hand sanitizers should be used only when there is no water and soap. You can simply make your own DIY hand sanitizer that's safe and efficacious at residence, and then use whenever you're out there.

In my particular instance, you will find yourself in need of daily use of the hand sanitizer. when there's no water and soap approximately, children mostly would like to snack, and once they snack, we might have a snack too. So, that's one of those factors we have to carry with us always.

Methods for this hand sanitizer do not contain alcohol

because we don't want to use alcohol on our children. In this method the microbe-killing components are the essential oils. If you want not to use essential oils, you will need to change this formula to use at least 60 per cent of alcohol mixing.

Tip to keep your home disinfected

If you're searching for a house sanitizer, our go-to is Nature Energy, it's just as good as bleach but without the harmful chemicals. Force of Nature is registered as EPA for the disinfection and sanitization of health facilities, ICUs, daycares, educational institutions and more.

DIY Hand Sanitizer Spray

This method makes this one-ounce spray bottle sufficient to fill up. If you reuse an old bottle of hand sanitizer, you'll definitely need 2 oz of this method so just almost double product. Bear in mind that this recycle does not comprise additives so you should make or use it in small lots.

The recipes are made in about 1 minute.

Steps

INGREDIENTS

- 1 oz glass spray bottle

- 1 tablespoon Aloe Vera spray or Aloe Vera gel (after making this   recipe many times, I recommend using the Aloe Vera spray)

- 1 tablespoon alcohol-free witch hazel

- ¼ teaspoon vitamin E oil

- 30-36 drops of Germ Destroyer (get on Amazon)

- If you don't have Germ Destroyer, you can use 30 drops to tea tree oil and 5-10 drops of lavender essential oil

INSTRUCTIONS

This is such a simple recipe to make!

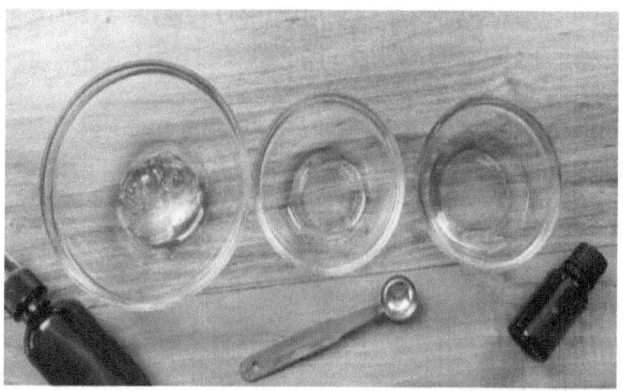

1. If you are using the Aloe Vera moisturizer, all you have to do is use a small funnel to put all the additives into the bottle. Then shake it and it's prepared.

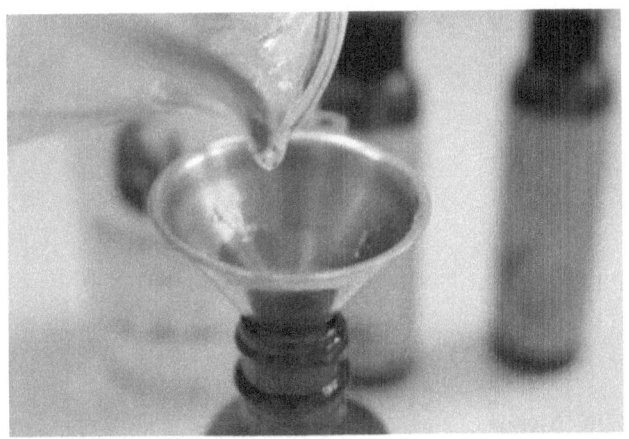

2. If you use Aloe Vera gel though, then you'll have to blend all the additives in a small glass jar.

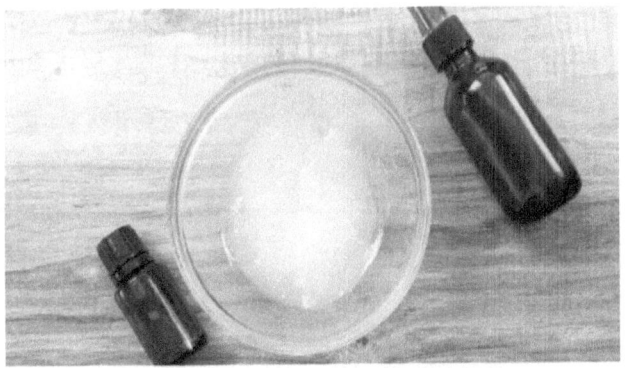

3. Mix them together well so that the gel coherence has become more liquid.

4. Move into the flask. Using a pipette, it is simple to pour it if you used the gel.

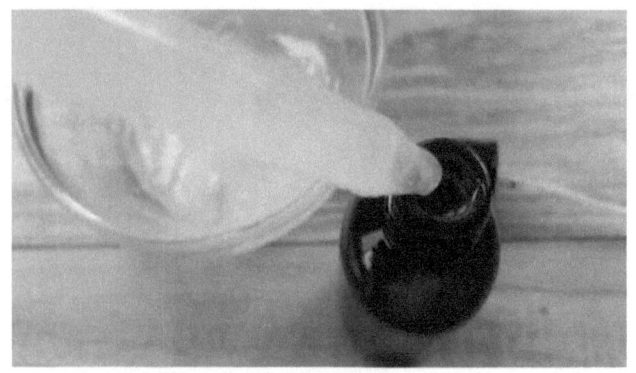

5. Giving it shake, and it is prepared! Spray as you would any standard hand sanitizer spray on your hands.

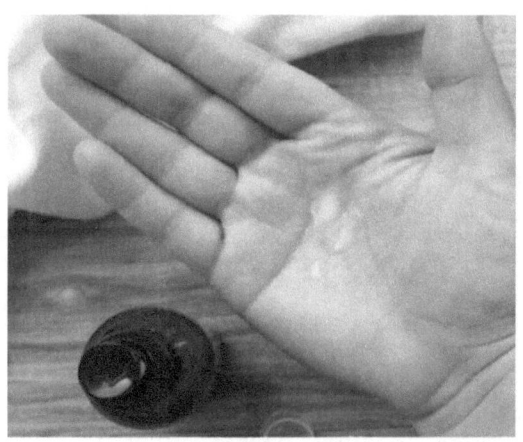

6. Keep it in your bag and use it, as necessary. Before any use do not hesitate to shake it. You will absolutely adore this recipe.

DIY Hand Sanitizer With Alcohol

As the virus pandemic started to expand, wherever feasible the Centers for Disease Control has suggested "social distancing" and self-isolation. And one consequence of that, as you may have realized, is things flying off the shelves at your local supermarket. One of those stuff? Hand sanitizer.

Remember what everybody is going to buy next — alcohol, aloe vera, and essential oils — and get ahead of the trend while you're going to stock up on non-perishables, drugs, and other vital things you may need in the next several weeks.

No, that's not the remedy for a trendy, boozy beverage, if you like, a quarantine. As individuals (namely, Googling) figure out how to make their own home sanitizer — know, hand sanitizer was the first thing people came after during the first virus initial attack! — Isopropyl alcohol, aloe Vera gel and essential oils are expected to be the next priorities for the communities. If you've been looking for DIY hand sanitizers, here's what you'd like to know — from theories to reality, to the advice of a specialist on how to make it yourself.

Are hand sanitizers effective and antiviral?

Next, it's absolutely justifiable that you want to know if it's successful before you go through the hassle of learning to make hand sanitizer at home. And perhaps most significantly if the virus is successful.

The Centers for Disease Control suggested ethanol-based (alcohol-based) sanitizers such as hand sanitizers as a means of preventing the transmission of virus in an official comment entitled, "CDC Report for Healthcare Workers on Hand Hygiene during the Reaction to the Global resurgence of virus."

"CDC guidelines illustrate the essential role of hygiene practices in avoiding pathogens from spreading to a wide variety of pathogens in healthcare settings," the statement says. "The potential of hand hygiene, especially hand washing or the use of hand sanitizers dependent on alcohol to deter infections, is linked to decreases in the number of active microbes that peripherally contaminate the hands."

"Hand washing manually extracts contaminants although laboratory results indicate that 60 percent ethanol and 70 percent isopropanol, the active ingredients in CDC-recommended alcohol-based hand sanitizers, detoxify biologically-related viruses with identical physical characteristics to the 2019-virus," it adds.

The CDC has also suggested hand sanitizers dependent on alcohol as the "preferred method of hygiene practices in healthcare environments."

You would like to ensure you have 99 percent isopropyl or rubbing alcohol, Aloe Vera jelly, and essential oils such as tea tree oil, lavender, citrus, clove, peppermint, frankincense, thyme and/or oregano oil, if you'd like to make it at home.

Nevertheless, it is important to keep in mind that antibacterial is not the same as antiviral. Since the virus came into being, this may not be as good for other essential oils including antibacterial properties.

These all have antibacterial properties so I would suggest them. "Just note, this virus cannot function the same as other antibacterial agents." So, to be sure, while DIY home sanitizer is not suggested as a 100 percent security feature, here is the break down if you should try to make it.

What ingredients do you need to make hand sanitizer?

Hand sanitizer with three primary components can indeed be made at home: isopropyl alcohol (ninety-one per cent or higher), Aloe Vera powder, and maybe a few drops of essential oil. Now, until you mix all those items, there are some points you should learn.

Isopropyl alcohol is the principal sanitizing component in this recipe for DIY hand sanitizer. To keep your at-home sanitizer as safe as possible, keep sure you substitute alcohol that is up to or above ninety-one per cent alcohol. Optimally, the most you can achieve is ninety nine percent, but anything over 91 would also work well to dispose of bacteria and viruses.

Aloe Vera gel is available in most of the markets. Put it another way, if you have an Aloe Vera plant, you should break off a plant leaf and use it to cure (and sanitize) as its properties. Because of its moisturizing qualities it is also essential to the recipe; it prevents the skin from drying out. The alcohol in this manual sanitizer method will cause your skin to dry out without Aloe Vera.

There are some which you can use for sanitizer when it relates to essential oils. Though, tea tree is probably the most popular basic oil to be used for sanitizer. Tea tree oil has antibacterial effects as well as antiviral, antifungal and anti-inflammatory properties. Although work on whether the essential oil of the tea tree virus can effectively protect is minimal, it is assumed to fend off the microbes involved with acne, staphylococci, micrococci, Enterococcus faecalis and Pseudomonas aeruginosa.

Cinnamon is another basic oil that is suggested for producing a hand sanitizer. In certain species, cinnamon essentially "deactivated" the viral constituents.

If you're only trying to feel nice in your hand sanitizer, try using lemon, citrus, peppermint, or lavender. That essential oil you choose, 8-15 drops should do the method everywhere.

What else do you need to make hand sanitizer?

Among these three primary components, you'll also need a mixing pot, spoon, measuring cup and a funnel. Though these items are not essential, they definitely make the procedures of weighing and sanitation much simpler!

Steps
How to make DIY hand sanitizer

All is the ratio. The ratio that you need to the most powerful hand sanitizer relies on how much alcohol you consume.

For e.g., if you're using ninety-one per cent Isopropyl alcohol, you 're going to want a 3:2 ratio, 3 tablespoons of alcohol to Aloe teaspoons. When you use ninety-nine per cent isopropyl alcohol, you 're going to want a ratio of 2:1 (3 T alcohol, 1.5 T alcohol).

If you use ninety-one per cent of Isopropyl alcohol, toss 1 cup into a bowl and mix. Last, apply Aloe Vera gel 2/3 cup. Insert 8-15 drops of the essential oil of your choosing anywhere you want. Bring all together with a spoon, then use a funnel to turn the blend into a filled container.

If you're not using a bottle with a pump, you should insert your DIY hand sanitizer into a travel go-tube and one of those small salad dressing valves that you place in the meals for babies!

Alternatively, a spray bottle will work, too.

- 1 cup Ever clear

- 1/3 cup Aloe Vera

- 2 tablespoons of coconut oil

- A few drops of essential oil

- Hydrogen Peroxide (amount dependent on supply)

- Mix it up in a bowl and portion into a container.

What if I don't have Aloe Vera gel?

No problems, without the Aloe Vera gel you can still make a hand sanitizer. Only swap Aloe Vera with witch hazel. When you use the witch hazel as an option, the sanitizer 's quality would feel more like a mist. A spray bottle is probably much better, for that reason.

When you're nervous about washing your hands because of the alcohol, you should add 1/4 teaspoon of vitamin E spray, too.

How else to disinfect at home?

Thorough maintenance is one of the most effective measures that we can do to suppress the virus to avoid it spreading. This involves handwashing but also daily sanitization of our homes.

We should be disinfecting our house periodically as per CDC guidelines. "First and foremost, more than 20 seconds of repeated hand-washing is necessary. Using latex gloves, then wash disinfectant or soap and water surfaces clean. You have to wipe down of chairs, doorknobs, lamp switches, countertops, handles, seats, telephones, buttons, toilets, and sinks.

So, what's the most effective way to wipe down these surfaces?

You can also use 70 percent of alcohol to thoroughly clean surface areas. "You can use 5 T bleach and 1 gallon of water to produce bleach solution. Personally, if you have no alcohol or bleach, you will not consider doing anything to disinfect with any vinegar or baking soda.

After all, the most effective avoidance strategy of all may be simply social distancing.

The distancing from society is quite necessary. It's vitally important that everyone bear this in mind and pay attention.   "And our new health care system won't afford the effect of being ill at once... The reason we're doing this is we won avoid the transmission of the epidemic and ease the pressure on our new health care system."

DIY Hand Sanitizer With Alcohol (Fresh Aloe Vera + Vodka)

store shelves nationwide are cleaned out of hand sanitizer and basic ingredients for DIY models using Isopropyl alcohol, Everclear, and Aloe Vera/487 gel will be nowhere in sight- what to do? Here is another treatment that combines new Aloe Vera and any high-proof alcohol you can obtain.

This recipe is supposed to help those people who have no access to hand sanitizer, isopropyl alcohol, or Everclear. Most shops in city do sell aloe vera gel. A mist hand sanitizer-not a water sanitizer-is this formula.

It seems that many of us just want to know even at this moment we 're vigilant about our own wellbeing and self-care — this recipe is here to help to give us comfort, a sense of purpose and some germ-busting strength at a period when supplies are momentarily restricted!

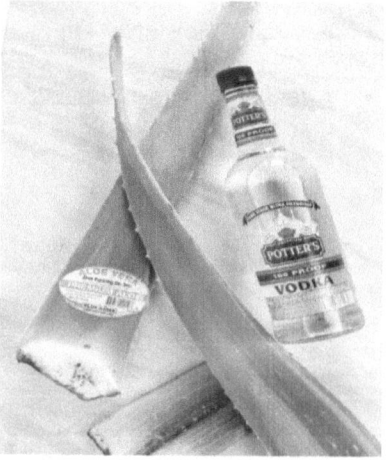

This fresh Aloe Vera hand sanitizer has the quality of a fine, sprayable fluid, not a gel!

HOW TO CUT FRESH ALOE

At most food products markets, Mexican markets, and restaurant supplies shops, a spear of new Aloe Vera is widely available for purchase. One stake of Aloe Vera yields around 1 cup of Aloe Vera gel and will remain in the fridge for 1-2 weeks: in the refrigerator for up to 3 months.

When you have ever fileted a fresh tuna, you'll be acquainted with the method of having fresh aloe. To begin with, fresh aloe can be gritty, slimy, and exotic - you'll certainly want a large cutting table and a good knife. I considered a compact knife to be best to use, because you can operate with a sawing action.

Start at the aloe staple core which is the largest portion and also has a white or light color. Check for where the light shading will vanish and resume the green coloring and chop off the white section. Your initial look at the fresh, strange-looking Aloe Vera powder, isn't it?!

Now switch to the Aloe Vera 's top and thinnest section. The gel in the slim tip is available, with a limited amount of gel that require just more effort and maneuvering with the knife. Check for a location where the spear is roughly 1 "thick and cut. There may be a certain yellow sap dripping from the Aloe Vera. There can be a stinky scent, too. It's usual!

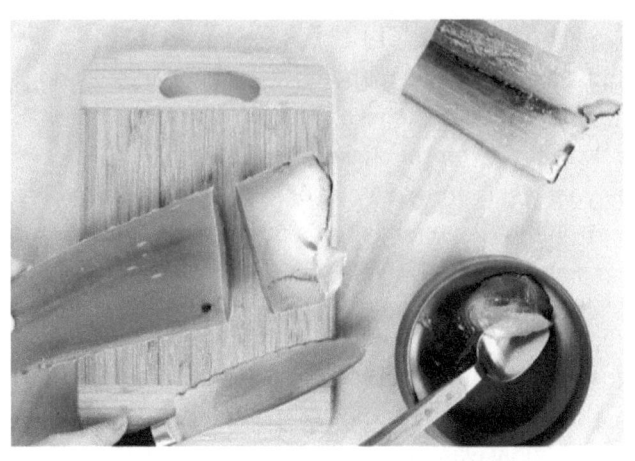

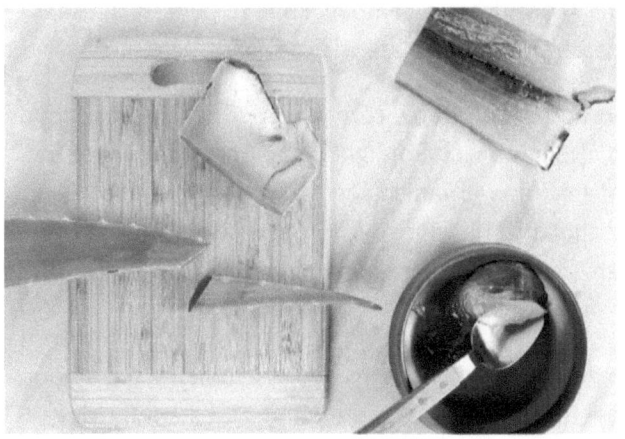

Now you'll be left with an aloe filet comprising of the plant's densest and most flavorful part — Here's how to get to the great stuff!

Switch the aloe on its side for a correlational view, starting from the bottom and largest end of the aloe. Position your knife as near to the edge as feasible, just below the outer green surface, and apply pressure or a soft stitching motion to hold the cut shallow. You can detach your knife after you've managed to make one slice and start softly peeling back the outer green skin. Proceed slicing as nearly as possible to the edge of the aloe filet and peel off the green skin unless you have revealed one part of the aloe entirely.

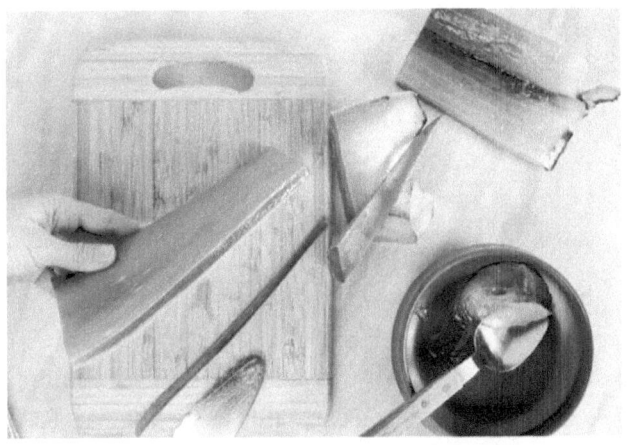

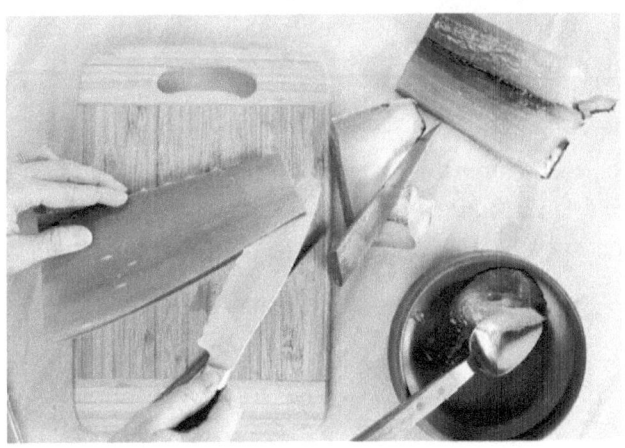

The best approach is to only use a spoon to scrap the green content off the Aloe Vera gel.

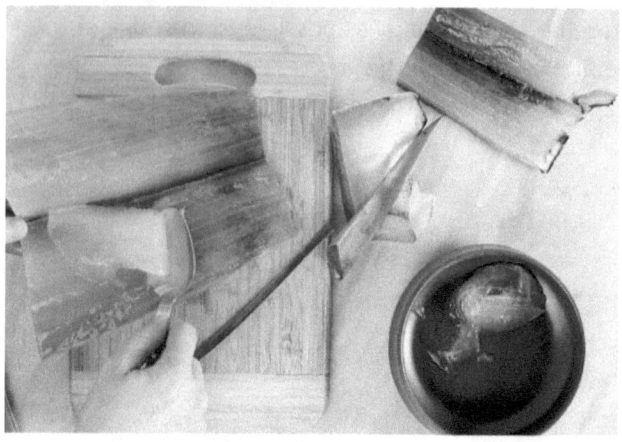

Place the aloe in a saucepan and wash off any yellow sap under cold water. For this recipe we will just require 1/4 cup Aloe Vera gel, you can easily weigh the part to mix and then preserve the remainder of the aloe in chunks to transfer to the smoothies or save for summers sunburns!

A reminder about frozen aloe, the consistency varies from frozen after the thawing. The gel becomes less rigid and waterier, it's barely noticeable in smoothies but it has a lighter, more watery quality for topical skin procedures.

Steps

HOW TO MAKE FRESH ALOE VERA HAND SANITIZER

To produce this fresh Aloe Vera hand sanitizer, we should mix the aloe to split it down entirely, then mix it with alcohol once again. For this method you can use a mixer, food processor, or bullet style blender.

Isopropyl alcohol is the ideal disinfectant to be used to make a hand sanitizer with homemade Aloe Vera-it has an alcohol concentration of ninety-one per cent. Secondly, a highly tested grain alcohol like Everclear- will be seventy five percent -ninety five percent alcohol. Because most cities and grocery stores are presently out of the above products, you should use high-proof vodka (or other alcohol) as an alternative, ideally with alcohol of sixty five percent -seventy-five per cent.

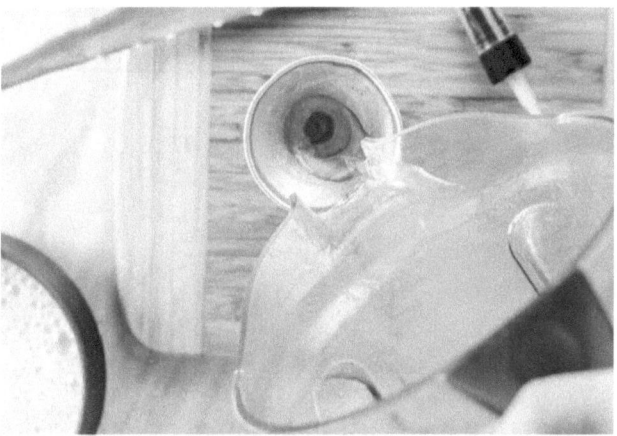

Here's the skinny: Hand sanitizer requires at least sixty

percent of alcohol to be approved by the CDC to be safe. A sixty per cent alcohol, calls for high-proof vodka, right? True- when we dilute the vodka with Aloe Vera gel, this sanitizer is going to drop below sixty per cent. Using a fifty percent vodka with alcohol may further reduce the amount of alcohol. Make logical sense? What should you do? This recipe is aimed to assist those people who have no significant exposure to hand sanitizer, isopropyl alcohol, or Everclear. Most shops in our city do sell Aloe Vera gel.

DIY SANITIZER ALCOHOL PERCENTAGES

The given table is an approximation focused on the

alcohol evidence used for the ultimate percentage of this hand sanitizer formulation. This is only an estimate, which can't be assured.

Base Alcohol %	Fresh Aloe Vera	Alcohol	Final Estimated Alcohol %
80 proof 40%	1/4 cup	3/4 cup	30%
100 proof 50%	1/4 cup	3/4 cup	38%
120 proof 60%	1/4 cup	3/4 cup	45%
151 proof 75%	1/4 cup	3/4 cup	56%
Isopropyl Alcohol 91%	1/4 cup	3/4 cup	60%
190 proof 95%	1/4 cup	3/4 cup	64%

CDC RECOMMENDED ALCOHOL PERCENTAGE

To order to safely remove germs and bacteria, the CDC suggests hand sanitizers be at least sixty per cent alcohol. Does a sub-60 per cent manual sanitizer harm germs, bacteria, and viruses? While this mix might not be as powerful as a sixty per cent hand sanitizer, it also has a high alcohol content.

That combined with the mechanical method of rubbing hands together through 20-30 seconds after application can also assist in removing microorganisms.

This DIY Aloe Vera hand sanitizer wasn't evaluated in the laboratory, I'm not a physician and I can't give medical advice. This is beyond range for the median household to evaluate the alcoholic content of the homemade hand sanitizer. (What do we say about the lack of research now?) Use this at your own choice.

Remember also: Improper use of hand sanitizers or handmade hand sanitizers that may have a concentration of alcohol greater than the average sixty percent, can have a rubbing impact on your hand. This can directly benefit, microscopic cuts and/or bruises on your hands possibly providing a microorganism point of entry.

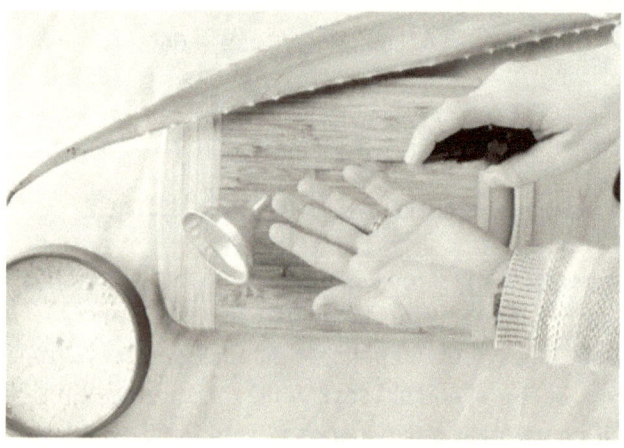

Hand washing is preferred overusing hand sanitizer!

Washing your hands for 20-30 seconds with soap and hot water is an efficient way to reduce the number of pathogens existing in our hands. We still do have handwashing, with or without a hand sanitizer, as an alternative to hold pathogens at bay!

Take priority of hand washing during hand sanitizer use, and make sure to moisten the hands after using hand sanitizer daily.

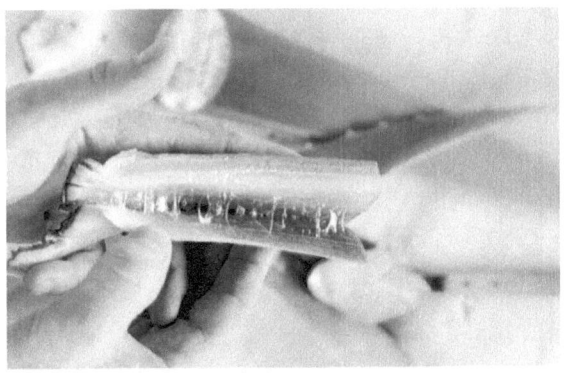

BENEFITS OF FRESH ALOE VERA GEL

Using fresh Aloe vera to produce your own Aloe Vera gel will make sure you get the decent things! When used medicinally on the skin, fresh aloe is admired for its hydrating moisturizer, cooling, and soothing effects.

That is included in the recipes of DIY hand sanitizer as its moisturizer qualities can help counter the drying that can impact high intensity alcohol on the hands.

Reading beyond the glossy front-facing logos and researching the panel of components to figure out the facts of what's really in a material is a custom that, sadly, we 're now getting more used to. Aloe Vera gel sold in supermarkets is another excellent example-most Aloe Vera product offered in shop shelves today contain various refined, organic, and preservative additives, with a relatively small percentage of real Aloe Vera for certain brands.

FRESH ALOE VERA + VODKA HAND SANITIZER

For DIY hand sanitizer recipes, fresh Aloe Vera and vodka can be a substitute when supermarkets are out of all traditional ingredients. This recipe gives you the choices to find your own hand sanitizer using away from the traditional recipes!

INGREDIENTS

- 3/4 cup grain alcohol

- 1/4 cup fresh Aloe Vera gel

- spray bottle

INSTRUCTIONS

1. Cut the Aloe Vera leaf at the root, the white part will diminish, and the leaf will be green. Generally, 2"-3" come from the leaf base.

2. Simply cut the upper portion skinny once narrowing to about 1" wide.

3. Cut the aloe leaf's spiny surface down the side of one side to expose the freshly gel within.

4. Place your blade carefully between the Aloe Vera gel and the green skin as you filet a steak, holding your blade close to the green skin. Put the knife just below the green skin before you approach the other side of the blade.

5. Drop the knife, then pull the green skin softly off. Begin to slice and peel until completely exposed on one side of the aloe. Using a teaspoon to clean all the new Aloe Vera gel out and put it in a mixer.

6. Stand mixer for 15-30 seconds, before there are no foamy bits left.

7. Measure 1/4 cup of the Aloe Vera gel and the equivalent amount of isopropyl alcohol or grain alcohol after the label table. Merge the unique blend once again for 15 seconds to complete.

8. Load into a bottle of water, and stock for up to 3 weeks.

9. Spray on your palms for 20-30 seconds and rub palms together.

NOTES

The ultimate percentage of alcohol can drop below the CDC prescribed sixty per cent alcohol solution for hand sanitizer, relying on the grain alcohol utilized.

So much use of a hand sanitizer may have a negative impact on the hands. Wash your hands for 20-30 seconds with hot water and soap where feasible.

Method 1: DIY Disinfecting Wipes (Natural & Reusable)

These DIY disinfecting wipes make it easy to keep your home clean without problematic chemicals. They're easy to make, natural, and reusable — just wash and re-use! Our homemade cleaning wipes are made without vinegar, so they're safe for use even on porous surfaces like marble & granite. Read on to learn how to make your own disinfecting wipes with essential oils.

While store-bought disinfecting wipes can be helpful for instant cleaning, they certainly aren't environmentally friendly or effective for your breathing.

Making DIY disinfecting wipes with non-toxic additives such as vodka, castile soap and antimicrobial essential oils is healthier for gentle clean-ups.

Number of studies have reported that specific household cleaning items can in fact cause asthma or other respiratory disorders in otherwise healthy people, especially supermarket-brand sanitizing wipes.

In addition, the pollutants from several store-bought household cleaners may trigger an assault in those who already have respiratory conditions.

Undisclosed ingredients in commercial disinfecting wipes

To add to the ambiguity, producers are permitted to

retain customers in the dark on what precisely is in their cleansing products. Sadly, existing rules do not allow the listing of ingredient details on the product's packaging.

More and more cleaning product firms have suddenly started offering some product information on their business advertise. Though, those descriptions are also not accurate.

The Environmental Working Group site is a go-to for manufacturing companies are permitted to leave off their labels of the ingredient lists. The EWG also offers additional information to consumers — including the adverse effects and the rapid degradation of each ingredient.

Here's a comprehensive list of other famous brands and their products for commercial wash.

Even so, if learning about the harmful chemicals in cleaning supplies turned out to be fearmongering, or if you say, "but how can these handmade wipes disinfect my counter? "Well, tests have shown that the antibacterial, anti-fungal and antiviral properties of certain essential oils.

Top antibacterial essential oils for homemade cleaning wipes

Without all the bad side effects of store-bought cleaning products, the preceding essential oils (in no specified sequence) combat bacteria and household odors. This is worth remembering that essential oils are simply an addendum to the alcohol's sanitizing properties.

As long as the wipes formula also includes powerful disinfectants such as high-proof vodka (or rubbing alcohol), you can make disinfecting wipes with natural oils. Do not depend on essential oils as your primary disinfectant, particularly just after an effective epidemic of the virus.

Subsequently, you can replace any other mixture of antibacterial essential oils from this list with the essential oils used in the description below:

Essential Oils:

- Eucalyptus

- Lemongrass

- Tea Tree Oil

- Grapefruit

- Palmarosa

- Cinnamon

- Rosemary

- Bergamot

- Orange

- Clove

- Oregano

- Thyme

- Basil

- Lavender

- Peppermint

Unexpectedly, various studies have already shown that cinnamon is indeed the top performing important antibacterial oil.

Ingredients for DIY disinfecting wipes

In my homemade disinfecting wipes, I still use high-proof vodka which is a much more effective disinfectant. Vodka also serves as a non-toxic preservative that stops the fungus and microbes from developing. The alcohol level of the vodka brand you 're using for this recipe is very relevant, however.

The brand should be at least Seventy per cent alcohol, since this is the minimum percentage necessary to kill a wide variety of bacteria and viruses while sanitation. That comprises such bacteria as E. Coli and lipophilic viruses, for instance influenza.

Vodka brands which follow the high alcohol level requirements usually involve:

- Everclear – 95% alcohol or 190 proof

- Spirytus Rektyfikowany – 96% alcohol or 192 proof

- Devil Springs Vodka – 80% alcohol or 160 proof

- Good ol' Sailor Vodka – 85% vodka or 175 proof

- Balkan 176 – 88% alcohol or 176 proof

- Pincer Vodka – 88% alcohol or 176 proof

When needed, the vodka can be supplemented with isopropyl alcohol (or rubbing alcohol) in this recipe. Important to remember, though, that isopropyl alcohol is highly inflammable, easily absorbed through the skin, and in some individuals its fumes can trigger blurry vision and migraine headaches.

Isopropyl or rubbing alcohol is also extremely poisonous if drunk, whereas vodka (or ethyl alcohol) is suitable for human consumption. Not like you're going to be drinking the wipe blend, so it's easier to use alcohol if you're trying to clean out places where little mouths are trying to be.

I recently saw DIY wipes vinegar and castile soap ideas

but combining vinegar with castile soap can cause the mixture to coagulate. The acidic vinegar and alkaline soap would also nullify each other leaving their washing capabilities worthless.

Consequently, vinegar is not suitable for stone countertops. So, if you have stone countertops, be careful of any vinegar-containing DIY sanitizing wipes recettes. That said, vinegar is already a good natural disinfect for several domestic items and is healthy.

Save money on cleaning wipes with reusable cloths

You can even save money by making these DIY sanitizing wipes because it is easy to wash the t-shirt squares (or cloths) used in this remedy and then substitute them in a corresponding batch. That also ensures these wipes are consistent with an environmentally sustainable, low-waste lifestyle.

you don't have any old t-shirts on hand or want a thicker fabric, relying on your choice there are still several types of sustainable cloths accessible. Heavy-duty microfiber fabrics, cotton towels and biodegradable bamboo cloths are only a handful of the available options.

How to use these sanitizing wipes

Before using your wipes, involve a combination of soap and warm water to carefully remove and scrub the area of any dust particles, grease, or sludge. Any soil or contaminants left on your surface can impair your wipes' sanitizing capability, and this is a big measure.

These wipes can be stored in your bathroom and kitchen cupboard for easy, light sweep up of germ-prone domestic surfaces. If ease is a plus for you, you could also use these DIY disinfecting wipes on the go, and you can convince them to be independent of brutal antimicrobial agents such as triclosan.

These wipes are also secure enough to be used on palms but make careful to use specific skin-safer oils such as peppermint, lavender, tea tree, and eucalyptus, and do not reach the mouth or skin upon use.

Even though, this should be mentioned that it is beneficial to wash your hands with soap and hot water. Even so, when you're not around a drain, those wipes are good than doing nothing.

DISCLAIMER:

Such cleansing wipes have not been checked in the laboratory to assess their efficacy towards viruses so kindly do not use them to this end. Each material used to cure viruses must have alcohol level of at least seventy per cent as required by the CDC as well as other medical associations.

Steps

DIY Disinfecting Wipes (Natural & Reusable)

Such handmade wipes wash and disinfect, without toxins, hands, and kitchen floors. Rather than brutal antimicrobial agents, made with vodka, castile soap and essential oils. No alcohol with an isopropyl! Environmentally friendly, recyclable, and non - irritating.

INGREDIENTS

- 1 cup high proof vodka

- 2 1/2 - 3 tablespoons castile soap

- 20 drops lemongrass essential oil

- 10 drops tea tree essential oil

- 10 drops eucalyptus essential oil

SUPPLIES

- Mason jar with cover or a disinfected container

- Old white t-shirt trimmed into pieces (or microfibers or other simple cotton towels)

- Sticky water-resistant label

INSTRUCTIONS

1. Squeeze the vodka into your mason jar.

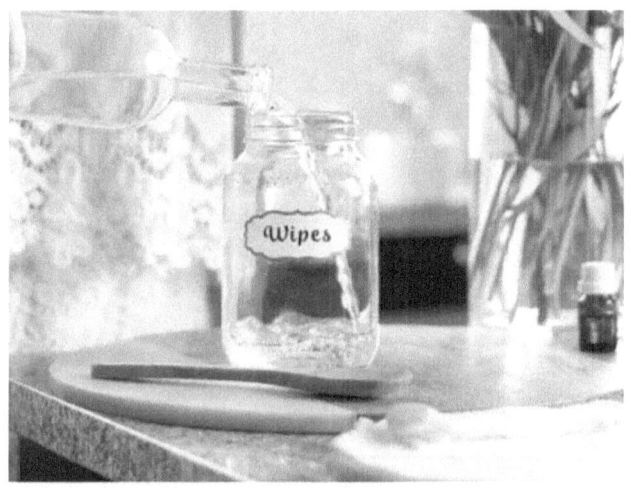

2. Introduce the essential oils that will quickly mix with the alcohol. Stir to mix strongly.

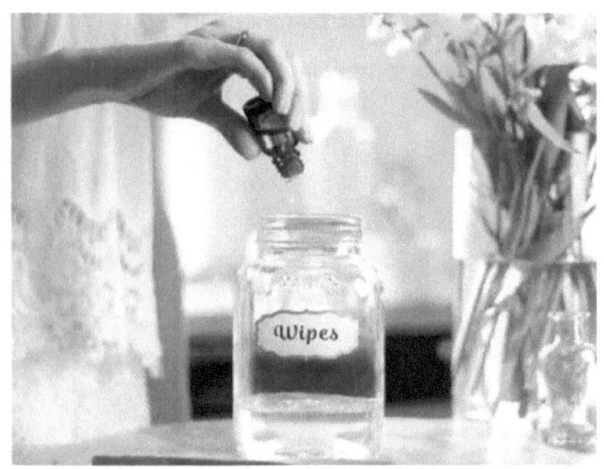

3. Introduce the soap, then wiggle it softly into the mixture. Make sure that trembling causes the castile soap to sudden.

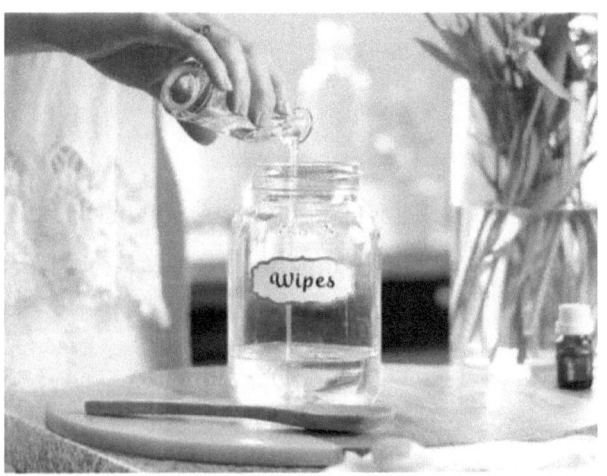

4. Wrap your cloths as is shown in the picture and put them in the container of the mason.

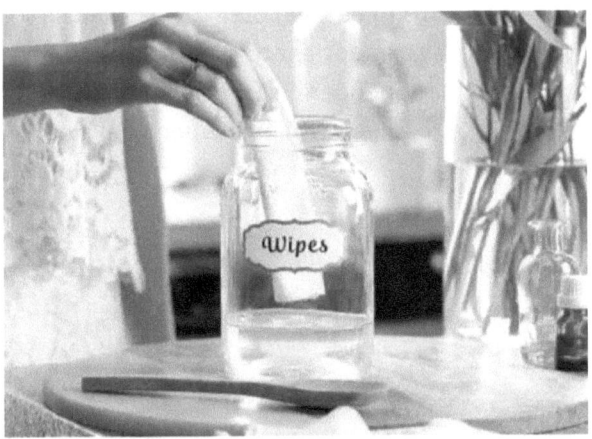

5. Replace the cap and gently swirl again so that the cloths get drenched with the solvent.

6. Keep the disinfecting wipes in a cool, dark spot, like under the kitchen or bathroom tap, with the cover securely closed.

Notes

If stored properly your DIY disinfecting wipes should last about 3-4 weeks. We don't advocate keeping items in plastic bottles or cans with large levels of essential oils. From all our DIY goods, we use glass storage boxes for essential oils, since essential oils are highly active and can leach contaminants from plastic containers. Please review your healthcare professional regarding the use of essential oils, particularly if you are pregnant or breastfeeding, have allergic reactions or have tiny kids in your residence. Other essential oils such as rosemary, clove, and eucalyptus to be used during breastfeeding are opposed. It is also important to avoid other essential oils such as rosemary, peppermint, oregano, and eucalyptus, or to use them with precaution with kids below 10.

Method 2: DIY Sanitizer Wipes at Home

Over the pandemic, sanitizing wipes became highly impossible to locate on the store shelf, but we need them more than ever to prevent getting infected. If shops are out of Clorox Wipes or Lysol Wipes near you, you can make your own disinfectant wipes at home, but you have to use the right recipes to make them efficient. The CDC has clear disinfectant protocols, and, in the pandemic situation, they are highly worth noting.

What ingredients work for disinfectant wipes?

Indeed, there are quite few other hygiene items that you can use to combat against virus in sanitizing wipes. Did not make it to shop or were online stores cleaned from what you want and need? This is how to get the most out of what you've got in your home.

Alcohol

You need at least seventy percent alcohol and in fact, that much 80-proof vodka is just 40 percent alcohol. Utilize booze that is at least 140-proof, such as Ever clear, Golden Grain or Spirytus Vodka, if you were to definitely raid your liquor cabinet for antiseptic reasons. Domestic rubbing alcohol is successful as long as it has an alcohol content of at least seventy percent.

Hydrogen Peroxide

Hydrogen peroxide can be used as a sanitizer as long as it is 3 percent — but retain it in a black or dark bottle, as the chemicals are unstable when get interaction to light.

Bleach, Lysol, Pine-Sol, and other antiseptic cleaning products primarily marked.

Using bleach or Pine-Sol, and items of the Lysol type — be very sure that the container says it is a true antiseptic, because not all of these goods and their numerous varieties have sanitizing properties. Like bleach these items can be combined with water and dissolved. The best approach here is the ratio: You need five teaspoons (or 1/3 cup) of bleach per gallon of water, or four teaspoons of bleach per quarter of water for small volumes. Like other items, their tags provide a reference to the water-to-product antiseptic ratios.

What doesn't work for disinfectant wipes?

Use ingredients such as essential oils and other forms of "holistic" cleaner because they do not actively kill germs or pathogens. The white vinegar, vodka and lemon juice don't work anymore. If you want to add essential oils for scent, that's acceptable — just make absolutely sure you 're not depending on them in your product as the real disinfectant.

How can I make disinfectant wipes with bleach?

Here are the following steps:

- Hold and cut a roll of structurally sound paper towels in half (a bread knife tends to work very well for that).

- Blend with two cups of water at a spoonful of bleach.

- Place any pair of your paper towels in an airtight bag.

- Put one cup of bleach solution into each tub over each of the rolls, then secure it.

How can I make disinfectant wipes without bleach?

If you are using Lysol, alcohol, or some other disinfectant rather than bleach, just adopt the disinfectant dilution ratio guidelines for the solution given by their bottle. When using hydrogen peroxide, make sure that those bottles are used in which the wipes safely are in dark and opaque.

What surfaces in my home are safe to clean with disinfectant wipes?

You want to make sure that the solution you use with your wipes and disinfectants is suitable for the surfaces that you will be washing. Review your labels and be sure it will not hurt, strip, or smear your products, for bleach or other disinfectant cleaners. Usually, disinfectant wipes are best suited to most hard, nonporous surfaces. These usually include the below but can vary your own house and its equipment:

- Countertops

- Trash cans

- Doorknobs

- Faucets and faucet handles

- Cabinet handles and knobs

- Drawer handles and knobs

- Toilets

- Light switches

- Remote controls

- Steering wheels

- Gear shifts

- Refrigerator handles

- Oven handles

- Microwave door handles

What else should I remember when using disinfectant wipes?

If you are using some form of disinfectant soap, make sure to be in a well-ventilated place. If bleach is used to make your disinfectant wipes, never use them with ammonia or any other toxin. Also be sure to give your disinfectant wipes sufficient time to properly kill the pathogen on surfaces — if you're not sure how long you need, verify out the directives for the EPA and CDC here.

Tips

How to Prevent From Virus

Either or not you are stocked up on the sanitizer, the CDC recommends that:

Wash your hands regularly: Nothing really beats washing your hands with soap and water for at least a few minutes. Hand sanitizer — including the actual, skilled stuff — should always be used while driving, even when you are unable to wash your hands.

Stay at home: But for important visits outside such as visits to the supermarket or to visit the doctor, don't leave the house. In location, that is also called sheltering.

Stay at least 6 feet away from other people: This is termed as distancing from society. Holding the gap makes it impossible for the virus to leap by respiratory droplets from somebody else to you (or vice-versa).

Wear a cloth face mask outside the house: The CDC now recommends everyone wear cloth face coverings when out in public where you may be near other people. Read out How to Make a CDC-Approved Cloth Face Mask (and Rules to Follow) guide to learn the benefit of a mask and how you should wear it. Kids under 2 years old should not wear a mask, nor should anyone who has difficulty breathing or taking it off. Do not buy or hoard medical-grade masks, like N95 masks. There is a massive shortage in the country, and the masks are needed by health care professionals.

Avoid touching your face: The virus can be transferred into your mouth from your hands.

Clean and disinfect frequently touched surfaces: Do it every day, particularly if you leave things or individuals, or enter your house.

Is It Safe to Use Vodka as Hand Sanitizer?

There are a number of different methods out there where individuals have used alcohol to manufacture their own home-made hand sanitizer, particularly because during the virus pandemic it is in high demand. And, owing to the heavy demand, some distilleries also sell their alcohol to the hand sanitizer manufacturers.

So, while that might be accurate, you have to remember that in order to be fully successful, the hand sanitizer has to be at least seventy percent alcohol per amount, in that specific form. It's not always nice to just spill alcohol into your mouth.

There are vodkas out there that go up to ninety five percent alcohol, which will be successful, but much of the vodka you 're going to see is either twenty or thirty percent, which won't disinfect.